MONIC
CR

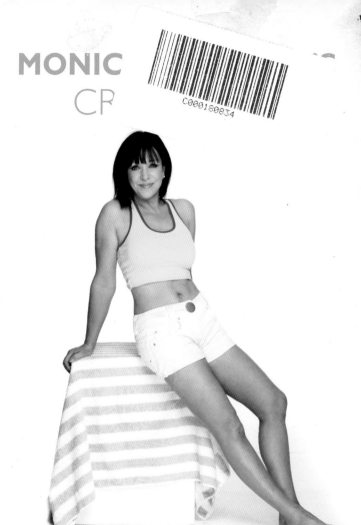

C000180834

... looking good is not a piece of cake

Photographs of Monica Grenfell © 2007 Mark Bourdillon
All other photography © 2007 Francis Balsom Associates Limited

Designed and produced by FBA PR & Design
www.fbagroup.co.uk

Printed in Wales by Cambrian Printers, Aberystwyth

Acknowledgements

To Charlotte
Hoping you will never need a crash diet

I would like to thank all the people who have made
this diet book a reality, especially Sonia Faustino at FBA Group,
Abby Knight and Christina Panayi who are just wonderful friends,
and all the test dieters who made it all seem such fun.

Foreword

Without being rich, young or naturally beautiful, you can still look stunning. No matter how your look is achieved, it has to start from discipline, from a sense of your own uniqueness, knowing your bad points and accentuating your good ones. Only you can know if you like your size, but the way you look and present yourself to the world reveals your attitude to life. It's a reassuring thought that even apparently flawlessly, effortlessly pretty women have figure problems. At least I have never met anyone, not even a model, who did not have something she wanted to put right. A small bulge here, or a few rogue pounds there are a cross most of us have to bear. Carelessly letting the pounds creep on, allowing your waist to billow and hips to spread, means you have let go of one of life's great pleasures: the satisfaction of feeling and looking your best.

Major lifestyle changes towards a better diet might be the best answer, but when the problem is small, a crash diet is a joy. It would be wonderful to believe that our shape and size are of no consequence and the only consideration is health, but we don't do things that are only good for us – we need other motivations. It is incredible to think that twenty or thirty years of happiness and satisfaction with your shape can be bypassed for the lack of a little willpower, and many women spend years in the misery of a weight problem they can't or won't address.

Pounds have a tendency to creep on. When those pounds reach double figures, getting rid of them becomes a chore. Sad to say, it is often a matter of carelessness, rather than the diet itself. Then of course, the problem of shifting them is daunting. It's far better, I think. to tackle the pounds as soon as they appear.

A crash diet is a helpful part of every woman's regime and women should never wear their diets on their sleeves, announcing to the world (dare I say boring the world?) that they have a problem. Far better to keep some mid-point in your weight so that a few pounds either way is not noticed and the enduring effect is "she's so lucky; she never puts on a pound." Only you know the truth of that statement!

In this weight-conscious world probably the first thing we think when we say 'diet' is deprivation and sacrifice. But there are diets for many purposes: diets for long-term everyday eating, diets for sports endurance, diets for diabetes or pregnancy. For most of us, the best diet is lifelong, intelligent eating: keeping meals low-calorie, getting out of the habit of sugar in coffee or mindless snacks. It does not mean never putting a spoon into a pudding. It simply means compensating at the next meal and using common-sense.

Crash diets might have had a bad press but they are practical and let's be honest, none of us is so famished that a week of restriction will cause harm. Crash dieting is merely civilised, a nice compromise between the pleasures of the moment and the pleasures of the future. You know you need to take steps by little signals; feeling uneasy in your clothes and bored with your look. You suddenly see the picture you present to the world and it doesn't fit with your idea of yourself. The effect of reaching this crossroads and taking the first step with diet comes from others, as they exclaim, "I wish I had a figure like yours!"

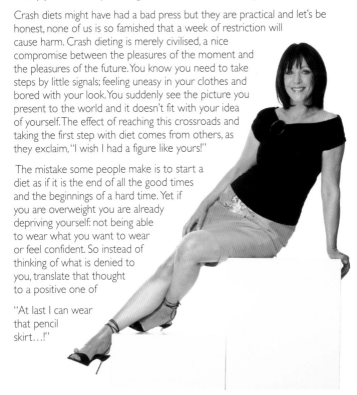

The mistake some people make is to start a diet as if it is the end of all the good times and the beginnings of a hard time. Yet if you are overweight you are already depriving yourself: not being able to wear what you want to wear or feel confident. So instead of thinking of what is denied to you, translate that thought to a positive one of

"At last I can wear that pencil skirt…!"

What is a crash diet?

A crash diet is a diet that restricts calories while not compromising nutrients. It achieves results by reducing energy so your body needs to dig into your existing fat stores and thus you lose weight. Fifty years ago, crash diets were all the rage. It is a fallacy to believe that women were more voluptuous and curvaceous, and diet obsession is a new fad: indeed, the fuller figures of the 1950's were a result of the gradual return to normality after wartime rations. With the restoration of food supplies, the propaganda machine went into action. It was a brave new world. A world of plenty. People were encouraged to enjoy food they could have only dreamed of during the six years of war. Milk, butter, cheese and cream were promoted for their 'natural' qualities and the same went for meat, bacon and eggs. Bananas, unseen for many years suddenly came on the scene again. Women's figures blossomed and the famous curves we all associate with the era were, in fact, an aberration. Women began to gain weight and they certainly did not celebrate the fact. Suddenly young women were cinching themselves into full-body girdles and long-line bras. Magazines of the era were jam-packed with special slimming breads, artificial sweeteners and biscuits and weird diets like the Gelatine diet.

I have a 1959 copy of VOGUE's NEW BOOK OF BEAUTY – SLIMMING AND HEALTH magazine, which was published four times a year for decades. In a feature entitled *New Ways to a Waist Line* it says

> *"Just now, with fashion at waist level, a lot of women will be interested in losing an inch or so quickly before they level out to an everyday plan that will maintain their leaner waist. Crash or fad diets are harmless for quick results, especially for quick pound loss in three to five days before some gala occasion. We know several models and actresses who swear by them. When carried out for a few days a crash diet is harmless to a healthy person – though it may be boring."*

I could not have put it better myself. Fifty years ago, you could not go shopping for another outfit the minute something didn't fit; money was in short supply and clothes bigger than a size 14 were unheard of for young women. On the whole it made economic sense to look after your weight and it was also not the done thing to ' lose your waist to a custard tart', as my mother used to say. This was the generation that invented extreme dieting. Three to five days of discipline is all it takes and I hope you will find my diets work for you as well as they worked back then.

Crash diets are brilliant for anyone with poor willpower. For these people, a slow and steady approach is useless. It might be desirable to lose weight gradually, but who wants to do that? It is like digging a hole with a spoon. But a couple of pounds weight loss is barely discernable when you have fifty pounds to lose. Dieting feels like torture. It is important to embrace the fact that slimming means you miss out on some things but you gain in other ways. Crash dieting gives good psychological weight loss and requires enough discipline to make the slimmer feel she is doing something positive – and this makes her keen to continue and not lose the benefits she has just worked for.

In the final analysis, our figures are the basis of great fashion. We all want to look good in our clothes. As a nutritionist, I know that weight gained quickly is usually lost quickly, given the right frame of mind and a reasonable attention span. This is how Crash Diet was born, to bring back the fun and the élan into dieting that says "yes, it's not ideal to diet and in many ways it's boring – but I would rather be bored than fat!"

Tried and tested

In the past eleven years I have been the health columnist for the country's two leading Sunday newspapers, the Sunday Mirror and the News of the World Sunday magazine. I have written a total of 563 columns of diet and exercise. I have written for numerous magazines both here and in America and have produced eight diet books. The diets in this book are the three most popular and asked-for diets from all those years. I still get letters about them. Of course, people kept asking "have you a book with this diet in it?"

The diets are intentionally niche. They rely on one or two key foods which compliment one another nutritionally, so if you do not like one diet the next might suit you perfectly. You can pass the book on to your friends to sample the other diets.

These are the diets and I am sure you will have great success on one – or all of them!

1 The Egg and Grapefruit diet
2 The Fruit and Nut diet
3 The Banana and Milk diet

Nutrition – the cornerstone of a good diet

Your body only requires nutrients in certain amounts. It does not recognise where those nutrients come from. Remember that people in other countries eat food very different from our own, food that will never pass our lips, and yet they still manage to thrive and lose weight. People get very hung up on the idea that they cannot lose weight because they hate fish or fruit or cottage cheese. This is nonsense. All that matters is that the body gets enough proteins, fat, carbohydrates, minerals and vitamins, from whatever sources, along with fibre and fluids for inner cleanliness. Whether you get your starch from a cassava plant or a potato is neither here nor there. So on these diets you have a balance of foods that provide what you need, and if there is a deficiency I recommend a supplement.

Here are the basic nutrients we all need for a good diet. I have included all these nutrients in your Crash Diets, so your health will not suffer even though calories are reduced.

Carbohydrates

The body relies on carbohydrates for quick energy. I must emphasise that carbohydrates aren't essential to the functioning of the body, they are simply very good at providing quick, efficient energy mostly because of the economic way they use oxygen for their metabolism. Excess carbohydrates are converted to fats to be distributed round the body as storage for leaner times!

The crash diets contain carbohydrates in the form of fruit, milk, yoghurt and vegetables.

Fats

Fats provide two and a half times the energy of carbohydrates but their energy can't be metabolised quickly. Fats are essential to the body, but because of their high calorie content, they must be eaten sparingly. As always, too many calories will turn to fat and unlike muscle, fat is dead weight. These diets contain fats in their main ingredients nuts, eggs and milk.

Proteins

You would not die if you did not eat carbohydrates, but you would die without protein. Proteins are essential because they build cells and repair our bodies. All these crash diets contain plentiful protein so whichever diet you choose you will have the right amount your body needs for health, maintenance and repair.

Very low calorie diets - the effective way to lose weight

Our bodies are feeding machines. Some people claim that the best diets are low-fat or glycaemic index or high protein, and I have read endless, ill-informed articles proclaiming that the only way to burn fat and boost metabolism is to cut carbohydrates. This is not true. The only way to lose weight through diet is to cut calories to fewer than your body needs. Some people lose weight the exercise method, eating a reasonable daily amount and burning several hundred calories a day in exercise. There is something to be said for this, but too much exercise has other downsides, like wear and tear on joints and muscles and stressing the body so the brain thinks you are running from danger. It is never a good idea to exercise for hours on end simply to use calories. Far better to do a half-and-half method, where you do moderate cardio every other day then tone and stretch for shape and firmness and eat a few hundred calories less than you need. As long as your body is fed and nourished, as it will be in your Crash Diet, you have no need of more calories.

Your questions answered

How much weight will I lose?

My test slimmers lost an average 7lbs in a week and 4-5lbs in the first three days. If the weight is of the stubborn-bulge variety, and has been plaguing you for some years, it might go from where on the body it chooses – usually the places that don't get disturbed, such as the hips and abdomen. Exercise always helps, but I am confident that you will love your weight loss and will feel and look far healthier and lighter than you have done for a long time. Fluid is held within fat and if you have been constipated, you will lose fluids as your system clears and feel magically lighter. Please don't listen to any of that nonsense about dehydrating and starving: if you have fat to lose you certainly won't starve.

I am worried about feeling hungry all the time

If you have been used to a bad diet with lots of stodge, you are bound to notice the change in food intake. But this is like anything: a change of pace in a new job, a change of air on holiday; a change in time zones or temperature… you can't ignore change and you will feel it. But do remember what I said about looking at the positive side: instead of thinking of what you can't do and what you are missing, remember that you have been missing out on a lot of things while you have been overweight. You have been deprived of confidence, self-assurance and pride in your figure. Instead of being worried about being hungry, try to feel bright about moving nearer to the day when you can zip up the dress again and feel it thrillingly loose around your waist. After a few days on your crash diet you will acclimatise to your new way of eating and trust me, your body will thank you for it and you will wonder how you ever managed to eat all that stodge before.

What if I don't like something on the diet?

If it is one of the main elements, like bananas in the Banana and Milk diet, or nuts in Fruit and Nut, this is the wrong diet for you. Slimming is not meant to be torture and you should enjoy it as much as possible.

What can I snack on if I get very hungry?

Hunger is only a sign that your stomach is empty. It does not mean your energy supplies are empty, as energy is stored in the liver and muscles and remains there for some considerable time; long after your stomach is empty.

I always recommend trying not to snack as this is a bad habit. Mealtimes should be enjoyable and an occasion. You should be aware of your food, conscious that you are feeding your body and enjoying the feeling of doing the right thing. Make meals colourful and enticing: a salad is one of the most attractive meals there is.

I sometimes get dizzy and light-headed when I go too long without a snack – this really worries me.

This is a natural reaction, cause by the release of adrenaline when your blood sugars get low. Blood sugars go up and down all the time. When we get very low, however, when we are hungry, your brain sends a signal to release fat cells into the bloodstream to provide emergency energy. Briefly, you might feel light-headed but many people feel quite normal. Don't imagine your 4pm slump or feeling tired all the time is necessarily helped by eating extra food. Sometimes this is true, but mostly, it's not. Energy from food does not necessarily make you energetic; it simply gives you the potential for being energetic. It is like filling your car tank with petrol and then leaving the car parked outside. The car has the potential for travel, but the crucial factor is the driver. Feeling energetic, I would suggest, is a state of mind and if you are feeling dull, depressed, anxious or bored, no amount of 'energy food' or calories will make a jot of difference.

As long as you are in good health, this should not be a problem. Of course, if you are worried you must see your GP straight away. I feel sure the light-headedness will wear off very quickly. If not, try a glass of skimmed milk or just a cup of tea or coffee with milk.

Tell me, Monica; do you diet?

Yes of course I do - I have a diet and its purpose is to keep me slim and healthy. There are not many women who would spend money on nice clothes and run the risk of not fitting into them. To feel the buttons straining and everything showing would be a feeling I dislike intensely. I'm not fanatical, but the right amount of effort to keep everything slim, firm and toned is worth it and no woman who considers herself organised and successful should find her diet a mystery or a chore.

I certainly crash diet now and again. I love the freedom it gives me. Far from feeling obsessed, crash and restricted dieting releases you from that endless poring over recipes, wondering what on earth you can eat tonight. As long as the diet is nutritious, you really have nothing to lose.

Should I weigh myself each week?

Yes, you should. How else will you know if you have gained weight? It is not always possible to know until you have seven or ten pounds on your frame, and then it is easy to get depressed and give up. Weigh yourself once a week, write it down and if you are a little heavy for more than two weeks, do your Crash Diet for a couple of days.

Always keep tabs on your weight. It is no more obsessive than checking your hair daily, looking for spots or tweezing your eyebrows.

It also means you can take steps when you have a tiny problem, rather than a big one. I suggest you record your statistics on the next page, as we all forget what we weighed and you can keep tabs, not just on this diet but the weeks and months ahead.

Your personal statistics.

Week 1

Date ....

Weight ....

Bust .... ins/ .... cms

Under armpits .... ins/ .... cms

Waist .... ins/ .... cms

Hips .... ins/ .... cms

Navel .... ins/ .... cms

Top of R thigh .... ins/ .... cms

Top of L thigh .... ins/ .... cms

Week 2

Date ....

Weight ....

Week 3

Date ....

Weight ....

Bust .... ins/ .... cms

Under armpits .... ins/ .... cms

Waist .... ins/ .... cms

Hips .... ins/ .... cms

Navel .... ins/ .... cms

Top of R thigh .... ins/ .... cms

Top of L thigh .... ins/ .... cms

A word about motivation

Motivation has been hard in recent years because of the barrage of anti-diet press and praise of bigger, fatter, more curvaceous figures. Now however, your motivation will get a helping hand I hope, because recent research into the causes of cancer have revealed overwhelming evidence that being slightly thin, with low bodyfat, will protect us from at least six forms of cancer. And despite the media's endless insistence that there is pressure to be size zero (UK size 4) how many people do you know who are very underweight? I have been a nutritionist for a long time and have personally met about three women who are a size 4. There is a saying that goes "those that can, do, and those who can't, criticise." Many critics of slim figures and crash diets are overweight themselves and resent the success of others. So please, refuse to allow yourself to be sidetracked. It is now official: it is healthier to be on the thin side.

Never be ashamed of being overweight however: whatever you weigh today, you will never be this weight again. Tomorrow and the day after and the next day, will all contribute to losing a few more ounces and they all add up. Soon those ounces become pounds.

Starting a diet and staying with a diet are different things, however, and this is where **determination** and **discipline** come in.

Many people will tell you that you look fine as you are, even though you know that you're unhappy with your size. But just because they sympathise, doesn't mean they understand. This constant fighting with your true feelings is stressful and upsetting. My advice is to listen to your inner voice. In the final analysis, an adult woman's bodyfat should not be higher than about 28% and although you feel healthy, if you are higher than this, we now know that this is not healthy. Unfortunately, no amount of bravado is going to change this.

Crash dieting is important for the body and the mind. Losing a few pounds is thrilling and tells you it's possible. Most of the testers wanted to stay on their crash diet either for a few weeks or for three days every week. They enjoyed the freedom from decision-making and enjoyed feeling disciplined. Whenever you want to give in, remember how you feel when you do. I have never met anyone who ate a massive dinner, three times what they really needed, and felt better the next day. I have never met anyone who waved away the pudding and woke up next day sorry.

Golden rules

1 Never eat thoughtlessly.

2 Never eat walking along the street, in the car or at your workplace (Desk).

3 Eat at designated mealtimes.

4 Eat at a table, using proper cups, glasses, plates etc.

5 When you have finished your meal, however small it was, clean your teeth, wash your hands and signal that your meal break is now over. You should not be tempted to eat outside these times (at any time, not just on your Crash Diet).

the DIETS

How to manage your Crash Diet

Do not rush out and buy half the supermarket. Obsession with food is a bad thing, and it is possibly what brought you to this place. Instead, the first thought should be 'I'm free from all that expense and all that shopping!'

Try and put the whole idea out of your head. Relax into your diet. You normally reach without a care for the cereal packet, so reach for the grapefruit or the omelette pan instead. This is only for a few days.

Try to be rigorous. Don't start adding a little extra dressing here or an extra tablespoon of something there, just because a few days have elapsed and your waistband is feeling loose. You need to be firm and focussed.

Substituting one food for another

Most people will have some problems. You might not care for shellfish, for example, or be able to eat it. Tomatoes might disagree with you. You might find chicken unpalatable or white fish bland. What I would say is, never give up or change anything simply because you find it dull or tasteless: you can add seasoning and let's face it, exciting, tasty food might be what got you to this place. I do see the problem, however, when you cannot eat something, for example being allergic to prawns.

If this is the case, I would ask you to exercise sensible caution and look for a dinner you can eat. The menus in all three diets are strictly calorie controlled, so you will still lose weight. Just make sure to keep the basic elements in place, which usually means eating the correct breakfast and lunch for your chosen diet.

Swapping between diets

I do not recommend swapping between diets because it becomes chaotic. Stick to one plan for three days and if you want to change, this is the point to do it.

Supplements

The diets are sound. However, as food intake is generally greatly reduced from what you may be used to, I recommend you have the following every day:

* 1 multivitamin tablet with iron or a good iron tonic
  (ask at the pharmacy)
* Omega 3 and 6 fish oil tablets

Exercise

Exercise is a vital component of any woman's life, and you will use more calories if you do exercise. I do not want you burning energy as if there were no tomorrow, so you should concentrate on figure-firming and streamlining moves. I will talk a little about this later in the book.

Now on to the diets;